Taming Idiopathic Toe Walking

A Treatment Guide for Parents and Therapists

Ileana S. McCaigue, OTR/L

TAMING IDIOPATHIC TOE WALKING

DISCLAIMER

Each child with which this tool is to be implemented should be evaluated regarding their general level of sensory integration prior to beginning the use of sensory strategies. This is done in order to determine the sensory area where the child is most likely to respond favorably as indicated by the clinical observations that relay the sensory areas of most need.

The sensory strategies listed in this manual are examples of possible solutions that have worked in this author's past experiences with children who displayed toe walking sensory-seeking behaviors with sensory processing disorders as a subcategory of a variety of diagnoses.

The author is not responsible for any possible injuries, sensory reactions or accidents that may result out of the use or misuse of the materials from this manual. It is further presumed that the therapist recommending the activities for implementing this specific treatment tecnique has had prior training in sensory integration theory, assessment and treatment planning in order to utilize it with regard to safety precautions and signs of sensory overload. Physical limitations may also prevent the use of some activities that may be contraindicated, depending on the individual's disability. Use of equipment listed and the sensory strategies suggested should be done only under the supervision of a **trained therapist** or other provider that has been trained by the primary therapist.

Copyright © 2017
ISBN Number: 978-0999103913

Library of Congress Control Number: 2017909440
Handy Occupational Therapy Treatment Tools (H.O.T. Rx Tools), LLC, Suwanee, GA

All rights reserved. This publication was meant to serve as a home program and progress record or treatment log provided by an Occupational or Physical Therapist trained in sensory integration and neuromuscular rehabilitation. Therefore, no part of this publication, other than the HOME PROGRAM forms section [pp. 29-30 provided in English and Spanish] and pp. 31-41 may be reproduced or transmitted in any form or by any means, electronically or mechanically, including photocopying, recording or any information storage and retrieval system without written permission from the author.

For additional information contact:

Handy O.T. Treatment Tools, LLC
Ileana S. McCaigue, OTR/L
P. O. Box 1658
Suwanee, Georgia, 30024
www.HOTRxTools.com

ACKNOWLEDGEMENTS

A note of thanks and appreciation is extended to the children that were served using the Toe Tamers for their patience during the course of evolution of this treatment tool and protocol. Additionally, thanks is given to their parents and/or teachers for their follow through in the regular use of the Toe Tamers. Without their consistency and perseverance, especially that of Angela and Mike Land, the positive, evidenced-based results obtained could not have been possible.

To the reviewers of this book: Warmest thanks are given to Irma Alvarado, Ph.D., OT/L, and to Margaret Rice, PT, for their ongoing support and encouragement during all my endeavors. To my respected, former colleagues, Lee Axelberg, PT, and Jayne Berry, OTR/L, as well as to the very esteemed pediatric Neurologist, Howard Schub, MD, for their willingness and time given helping me complete this project that has been a long process, gratitude is also expressed.

Thank you, also, to Vivian S. Gammell for her assistance with segments of the still photography, and to Maria Rodriguez Zaballa, Ed.S., for her expert translation of the home program form into Spanish. Though we are both fluent, I would definitely trust her translation over mine!

Taming Idiopathic Toe Walking

Section	Table of Contents	Page
1	Introduction	1
2	Definition of Idiopathic Toe Walking [ITW]	3
3	Impact and Possible Complications	5-7
4	Traditional Treatments • Physical Therapy • Occupational Therapy Sensory Strategies Physical Therapy Techniques • Medical Management	9-11
5	"Toe Tamer" Alternative Treatment	13
6	Design & Fabrication of "Toe Tamers": • Items needed • Directions for Fabrication	15-23
7	Protocol for Positioning of "Toe Tamers"	25-26
8	Treatment Protocol for "Toe Tamers" • Home Programs in English and Spanish	27-32
9	Documentation • Wearing Records • Wearing Graphs	31-41
10	Case Studies	43-51
11	References	53-54

Taming Idiopathic Toe Walking

TAMING IDIOPATHIC TOE WALKING

1 Introduction

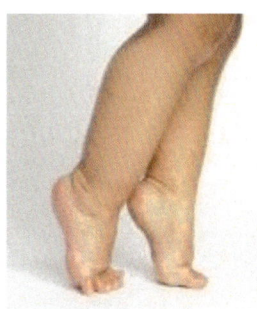

Toe Walking...

..is sometimes seen in typical children; however, it is very frequently seen in the children I serve with varying diagnoses. These include children with Autism Spectrum Disorder, Attention Deficit Hyperactivity Disorder of varying types, Specific Learning Disabilities, Developmental Delays and other disorders that are now considered to have Sensory Processing Disorders (SPD) or formerly Sensory Integrative Dysfunction cluster of symptoms as a component. Some children with Cerebral Palsy, Acquired Brain Injuries and other such diagnoses also display toe walking, but there is usually a known origin of involvement. However, the former group's underlying, root cause or origin has never been medically or scientifically proven, and is still considered hypothetical.

Having been initially certified in the administration and interpretation of the Southern California Sensory Integration Tests, as well as trained in the Sensory Integration and Praxis Tests and in the Neuro Developmental Treatment techniques, I have always approached toe walking for the SPD group as a sensory-based problem where the child or individual is visually or non-verbally guiding me to provide the needed sensory input. The original theory that the root of toe walking is a lack of integration of the positive supporting reflex from infancy, has the complication that the treatment for this theoretical basis is difficult to provide and measure. The sensory need for input is the basis for this therapeutic treatment approach which has been very successful for the majority, if not all, of toe walkers in my past experiences. I hope this treatment protocol for idiopathic toe walking is as beneficial for other parents with children that have this problem behavior, as well as for healthcare professionals who encounter this challenge in their therapy or medical practice.

Ileana S. McCaigue, OTR/L
©2017

TAMING IDIOPATHIC TOE WALKING

2 Definition & Causes

Toe Walking is...

Walking on the balls of the feet.

Idiopathic Toe Walking [ITW] is...

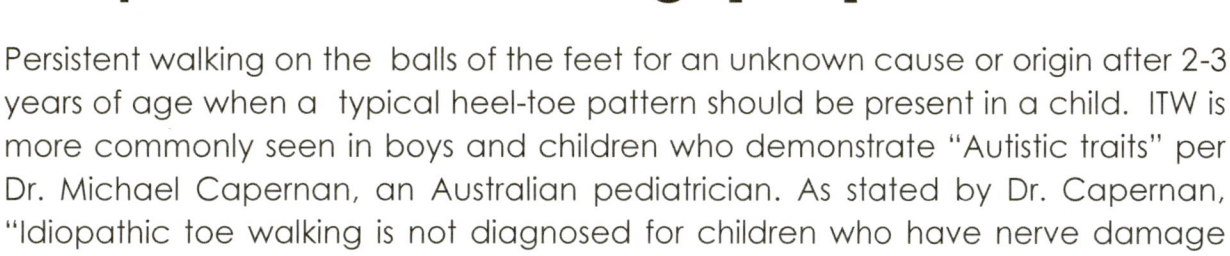

Persistent walking on the balls of the feet for an unknown cause or origin after 2-3 years of age when a typical heel-toe pattern should be present in a child. ITW is more commonly seen in boys and children who demonstrate "Autistic traits" per Dr. Michael Capernan, an Australian pediatrician. As stated by Dr. Capernan, "Idiopathic toe walking is not diagnosed for children who have nerve damage that causes stiff calf muscles or that occurs in children with Cerebral Palsy."

The cause of ITW is not fully known; however, the following factors can influence its development or persistence based on the theory that the root could be from a sensory processing disorder:

- Impaired tactile or touch processing (atypical response to touch sensations on bottom of foot)—could have a low threshold for hypersensitivity indicating intolerance for touch sensation/input;

- Impaired joint pressure or proprioception (sensing the body's position in space and joint awareness)—processing or the body's awareness of position in space could have a high threshold, needing atypical or above average levels of sensory input;

- Delayed vestibular processing (maintaining balance)—could be linked with atypical postural control or instability of the body's posture system, and difficulty performing developmental tasks such as hopping on one foot, squatting, standing with feet on floor, alternating climbing or descending stairs;

- Impaired motor control (control of body movements, large and small)—could be impacting balance and developmental skill development;

- Limited, specific muscle length and joint flexibility of the leg and intrinsic foot muscles—could enhance the degree of tightness of the downward position from the feet to the hips.

TAMING IDIOPATHIC TOE WALKING

3 Impact & Possible Complications

Idiopathic Toe Walking [ITW]...

Can be a neurological sign that should be assessed by a pediatrician, physiatrist, orthopedist or neurologist to differentiate between a true, neurological condition or a condition whose origin or etiology is still being evaluated. A child with sensory issues of an oversensitive tactile or touch system can walk on the balls of the feet to apparently avoid pressure that is difficult to tolerate on overly sensitive soles. This child displays walking on the smallest section of the feet with a typical "bouncing" motion to intermittently seek input via the balls of the feet. In extreme cases, the child walks on the back of the toes if the touch input cannot be tolerated on the pad of the tip of the toes. Over a long period of time, this persistent or "habitual" behavior, as labeled by Dr. Howard Schub, a well-known and respected pediatric neurologist, can lead to muscular tightness of the hips, calves and ankle muscles, as well as the small muscles of the feet. Consequently, shortening of the Achilles' tendon at the heel of the foot can occur making it difficult, if not impossible, to bend the foot back to rest flat on the floor for proper upright sitting.

As a result of the oversensitivity to touch on the soles of the feet, the wearing of socks and shoes is usually very difficult, and can become a problem in school or in the community. At home, a child that toe walks often prefers to be barefoot at all times, and tries to do the same elsewhere, tending to remove socks and shoes at the first opportunity.

3 Impact & Possible Complications

Idiopathic Toe Walking [ITW]...

One of the challenges of toe walking includes the child maintaining his or her center of gravity by altering his or her posture to accommodate for the forward weight shift. It is as if he or she is in a state of always attempting to avoid falling. In turn, this could alter a child's visual perception due to a visual field shift upwards and forward. This could also have a significant impact on a child's body sense or awareness. The bouncing on the balls of the feet from a constant need for proprioceptive or joint pressure input can occur while attempting to constantly weight shift to balance and maintain an upright position while walking.

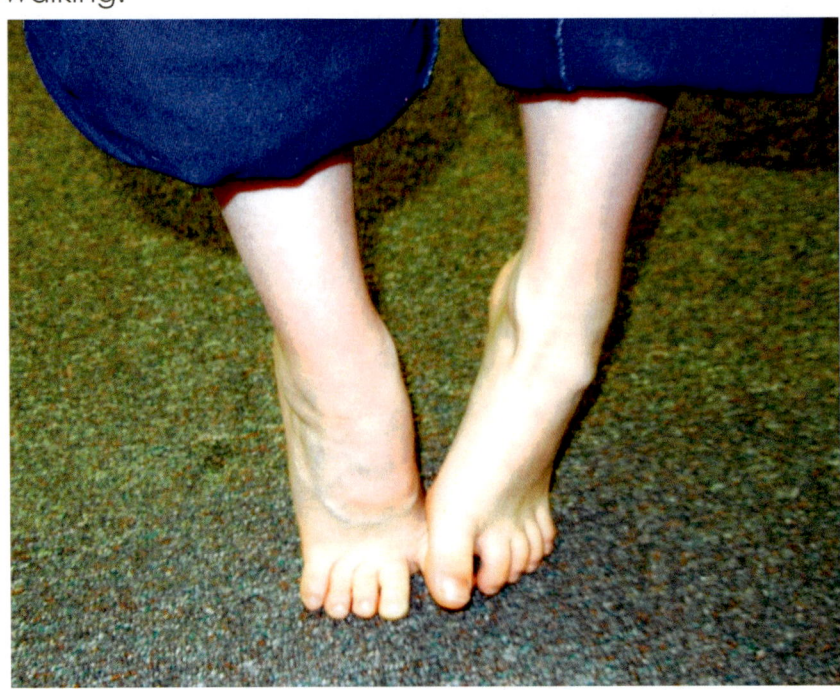

3 Impact & Possible Complications

Idiopathic Toe Walking [ITW]...

With a diagnosis of idiopathic toe walking, a child that toe walks past the age of 3 years old will be most likely able to overcome this behavior if treatment is initiated as early as possible. Based on theories of brain plasticity, the younger the child receives an intervention, the more quickly the brain can "flex" and develop neural pathways to overcome the atypical pattern of movement. The older the child or adolescent begins treatment, the longer it will most likely take to effect a true change in this atypical behavior. Through appropriate sensory input, a typical, age-appropriate gait pattern for walking with a full heel-to-toe follow through can usually be achieved.

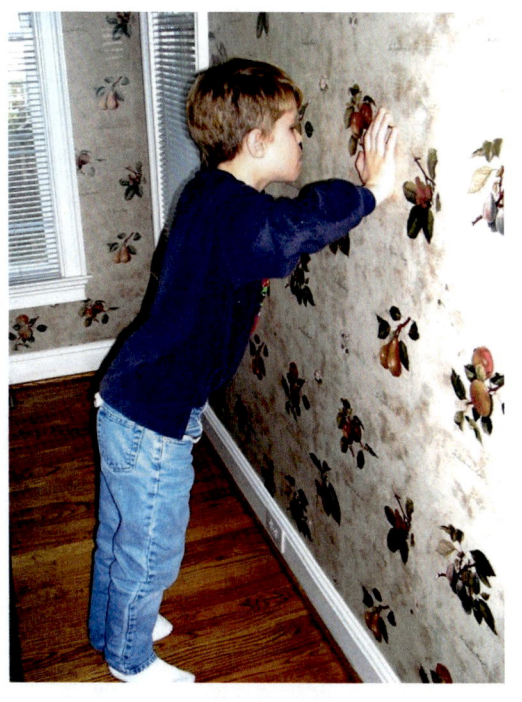

NOTE: This child's persistent, idiopathic toe walking resulted in a mild shortening of his heel cords. It further caused a limited ability to tuck his pelvis to straighten his back when performing wall push-ups. This position was one method to test for the possible impact on heel cord length. Another clinical observation, that could possibly indicate tendon shortening, would be an inability to sit on the floor with legs crossed at the ankles. This would require the child to pull the toes and feet back towards the body into dorsiflexion which would stretch the heel cords. This would be very difficult and often painful.

TAMING IDIOPATHIC TOE WALKING   7

4 Traditional Treatments

Re-Habilitation Management—Therapies:

A **Physical Therapist** may...

- Apply stretching techniques, and teach a parent how to properly stretch the heel cords to allow for stabile standing and upright sitting.

- Assess the proper fit of an individual's shoe to maximize the support for the insole of foot and ankle for greater stability and positioning of the foot overall.

- Recommend the use of specialized or high top shoes, as well as possible use of an orthosis. This could consist of a shoe insert or arch support, an SMO [SupraMallelolar Orthosis] just above the ankle or an AFO [Ankle-Foot Orthosis] that is worn between the knee and toes of the leg. These types of orthotics can be adjusted at times by the P.T., but are made by an Orthotist that specializes in the construction and adjustment of such devices. They are made to support alignment of the foot, which affects the pelvis and general alignment of the total body, and to keep the heel down.

- Suggest and recommend the appropriate amount of ankle weights to help push the back of the foot and heel towards the floor.

- Suggest gross motor activities to facilitate dorsiflexion or upward bending of the ankles, knees and hips to offset or counterbalance the toe walking position.

- Recommend or use modalities, analgesic gels or ointments and other treatments with a Physician's order if pain management is needed from complaints of tenderness or discomfort in the calf or thigh muscles, as well as the joints of the leg.

4 Traditional Treatments

Re-habilitation Management—Therapies:

An *Occupational Therapist* may…

- Provide a **Sensory Strategy Plan** via use of the **Scale of Sensory Strategies [S.O.S.S.®] Toolkit©**, to apply appropriate pressure and touch stimulation to the balls of the feet to help the individual meet the need for sensory input, achieving improved tolerance for tactually stimulating and weight-bearing activities. This might be accomplished by sensory strategies such as massage, brushing of the soles, deep joint input into the toes, and ankles, and/or use of vibration. Examples would be activities such as jumping on a mini-trampoline, hopping on two or one foot, sitting and bouncing on a ball or a ball with a handle, use of a coiled, pogo type stick for jumping with heavy input into the foot, jumping rope, etc.

- Construct or recommend the use of a weighted belt to provide input from the hips to the ankles to attempt to give input into the balls of the feet and lower the heel of the foot. One formula which has been used is to take 10% of the individual's body weight in a heavy medium such as sand, rice, metal washers, etc. to achieve the desired weight.

- Use a specialized brush to brush the soles of the feet with joint compressions from the toes to the ankles as part of a full body brushing program done on a regular basis during waking hours or with use on the legs only, depending on the therapist's orientation.

- Recommend the use of seamless socks or have the individual wear his or her socks with the inside seams facing outwards.

- Use shoe weights that are attached on the tops of shoes. They add pressure primarily into the sole or arch, not the toes or ball, of the foot.

- Collaborate with P.T. to design and fabricate soft, shoe inserts or soles to pad and protect the feet and toes with shock absorbing material.

4 Traditional Treatments

Medical Management of ITW:

A *Physician* may...

- Recommend Physical Therapy for exercises, stretching or modalities, and/or bracing if a child: 1) has difficulty with coordinated walking; 2) has stiff or tight calf muscles; 3) is unable to stand to weight bear flat-footed; 4) walks on the toes continuously past the age of 3 years old, and/or 5) has not met developmental milestones or lost previously developed skills.

- Recommend Occupational Therapy for assistance with the sensory seeking, sensory-based behaviors, self-help and/or developmental needs of the child or adolescent.

- Prescribe leg braces that support the foot and ankle, to maintain the length of the muscles and tendons as a preventative measure.

- Serial cast to correct an established and strong toe walker's tendency to stand on the toes which may have caused shortening of the heel cords, etc.

- Utilize injections, such as Botulinum Toxin to relax the heel cords.

- In extreme cases, perform surgery to lengthen tightened heel cords which would enable the feet and ankles to lower to return to a flat footed stance.

5 Alternative Treatment

This publication offers an alternative sensory strategy to the traditional construction of other low tech aids. The objective of these aids is to provide pressure to reduce or help integrate the tactile hypersensitivity that appears to impact gait, and result in atypical toe walking of unknown etiology or cause. However, the commercially available shoe weights provide input that is concentrated at the top or middle of the foot, as opposed to the ball of the foot or over the toes.

"Toe Tamers" described herein provide the needed input that the idiopathic toe walker seems to seek and need at a more exact location at the toes to facilitate a typical walking or gait pattern. The joint pressure or proprioceptive input is more intensely and directly driven over the balls of the feet from the top of the toes. This appears to relax or calm the need to plantarflex at the ankle or arch the foot in an upward direction. The bouncing action of walking on the toes can be interpreted as the child or individual seeking the needed proprioceptive input to override the intolerance of weight on the foot when touching the floor while walking or when flat-footed.

Additionally, though there are no accepted, scientific studies that utilize this strategy in the United States, some children respond very favorably to the use of intense or strong **magnets** placed in the same position as the "Toe Tamers". Each cell in the human body is polarized with a positive and negative charge. Magnetic energy is known to move fluid, air or other cells within the body when placed in close contact to a specific depth. Electromagnetic energy has an even stronger effect with greater depth of energy field to impact the body. However, it is not actually known how this input calms the foot area in some individuals to allow the heel to lower, and the ability to walk with a more typical heel-to-toe pattern. *Extreme caution is recommended with the use of magnets. They should not be considered for children or adolescents that have any implants, such as a Vagal Nerve Stimulator; a Baclofen, Insulin or any other type of pump; a pacemaker or any type of device that has a mechanical or electrical component which could be activated by the energy field emitted from the magnet.*

TAMING IDIOPATHIC TOE WALKING

6 Design & Fabrication of "Toe Tamers"

Supplies Needed:

♦ ***A pair of appropriately sized and fitting athletic shoes***

Athletic or sport shoes typically work best, especially medium to high top tennis shoes . The canvas or mesh type of these shoes offers support, but are flexible for ease of walking. They also allow the "Toe Tamers" to be best secured since they typically have rubber or non slip soles on the bottom of the shoes on which the rubber bands can easily be positioned.

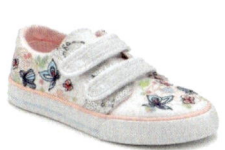 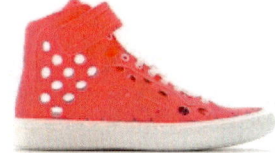 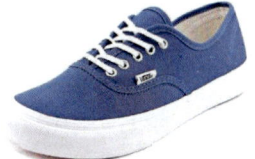 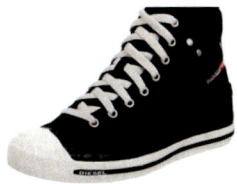

♦ ***1.0-2.5 ounce large, metal (steel) washers****

Check with local and/or online hardware stores for the range of heavy washers needed. [Example: 7/8 Steel Washers weighing 2.5 ounces each from The Fastener Center by Hillman™]

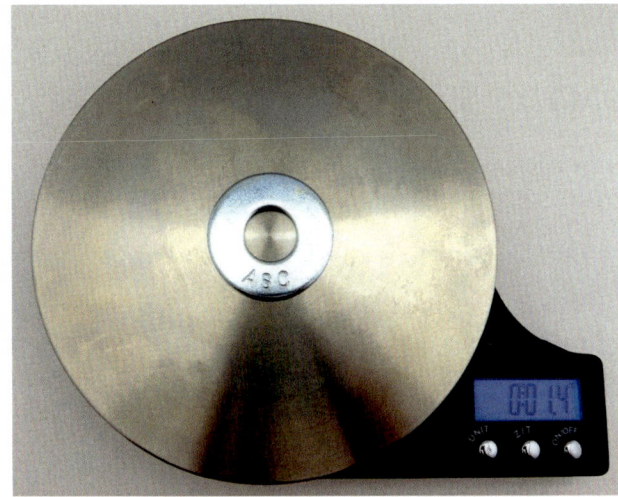 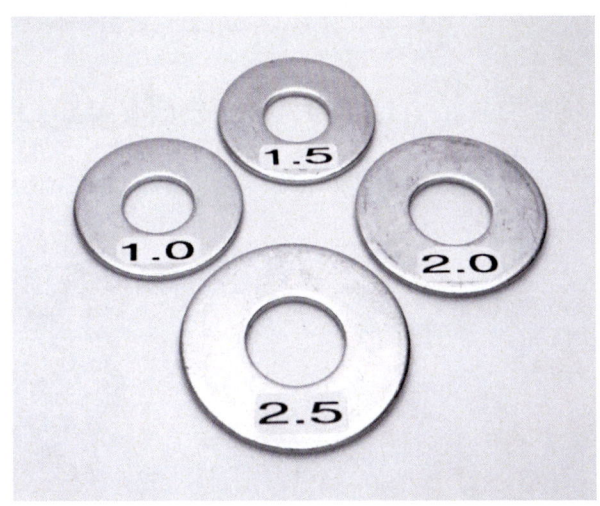

Digital scale used to weight washers.　　　　　* Weight values were rounded up.

TAMING IDIOPATHIC TOE WALKING　15

6 Design & Fabrication of "Toe Tamers"

Supplies Needed:

- **Duct tape or heavy duty, waterproof, adhesive, pliable, cloth-backed tape of desired pattern and/or colors**

    Have the child select the desired pattern and/or color of tape to be used to cover the washers. This is done not only to prevent the washers from slipping, but to protect the individual's shoes and feet from the metal of the washers.

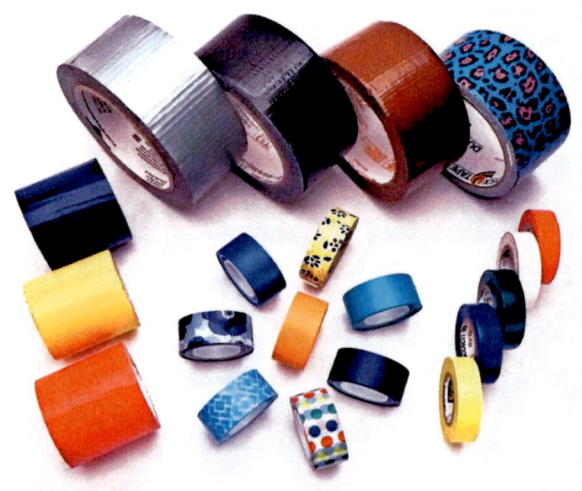

- **1-2 Super sized rubber bands**

    12", 14" or 17" size can be found at local and online office supply stores.

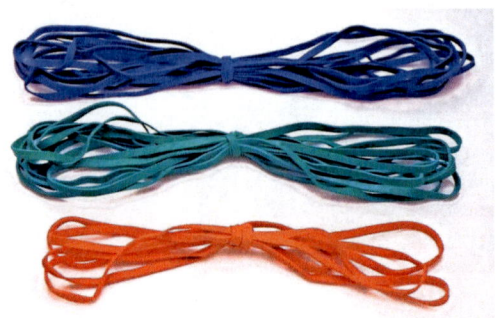

TAMING IDIOPATHIC TOE WALKING

6 Design & Fabrication of "Toe Tamers"

◆ Directions on How to Construct "Toe Tamers":

STEP 1 *Weigh the child without shoes.*

STEP 2 *Determine the washers needed based on the child's weight.*
The range of weights is 1 ounce per every 10 to 15 pounds of body weight. Divide the weight by 10 to 15 to determine the number of ounces needed for adequate pressure input directly into the ball of the foot from the top of the shoe.

NOTE: The weight range is 1 ounce per every 10 to 15 pounds of body weight.

To determine the amount of weights needed, complete the following formula:

- Child's total body weight ÷ 15 = Lower end weight
  to
- Child's total body weight ÷ 10 = Upper end weight

    [Example: 60 lbs. ÷ 15 = 4 ounces minimum
                to
             60 lbs. ÷ 10 = 6 ounces maximum]

Therefore, the total range of weight per foot = 4-6 ounces to achieve the desired impact.

Initially, use a combination of washers to equal 4 ounces of weights.
[Example: 2 X 2 ounce washers = 4 ounces of washers.]

If this amount does not calm the toes, then gradually increase until the desired weight is reached that facilitates optimum gait or heel-to-toe strike is achieved when walking.

[Example: Add 1 to 2 additional ounces in increments as needed, such as an extra 1 ounce weight or another 2 ounce weight until the desired effect (feet on the floor or typical gait pattern when walking and/or standing) is achieved.]

6 Design & Fabrication of "Toe Tamers"

♦ Directions on How to Construct "Toe Tamers":

STEP 3 **Select the number of washers** that would be needed to achieve the desired weight per shoe [3 X 2.5 oz. washers = 7.5 ounces per foot].

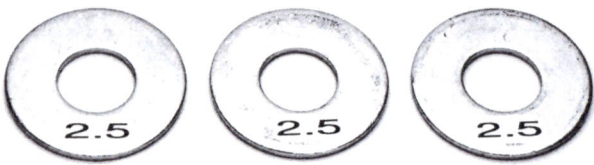

*Values are rounded up.

STEP 4 Then, **stack the washers** by arranging them in a vertical row to concentrate the force directly downward.

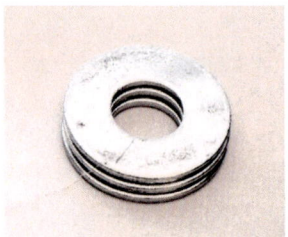

STEP 5 **Cover the weights** with duct tape or other type of strong adhesive material by wrapping them so they are completely covered to prevent exposure to the metal.

NOTE: Keep the center of the washers open so as to form a "tunnel" or tube in which to insert or thread the rubber bands.

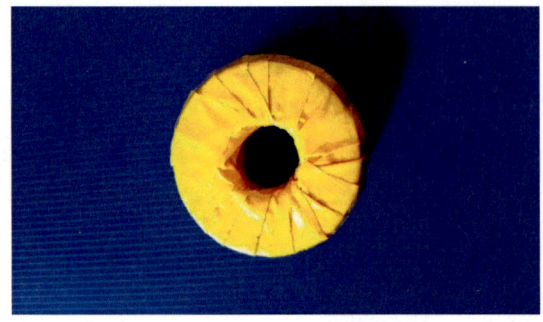
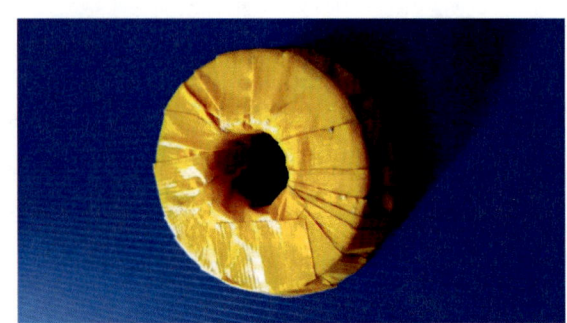

TAMING IDIOPATHIC TOE WALKING

6 Design & Fabrication of "Toe Tamers"

♦ Directions on How to Construct "Toe Tamers":

STEP 6 Once the weights are completely covered, select one of the rubber bands for each shoe to be used to secure the "Toe Tamers". The length used will depend on the width/size of the toe at the end of the shoe. Each band should be long enough to snugly wrap around the end of the shoe. Usually, the smaller 12" length is sufficient unless the shoe size is very large and wide.

STEP 7 Thread one end (A) of the long, sturdy rubber band through the center opening. Pull the end (A) through the washer opening one-half way.

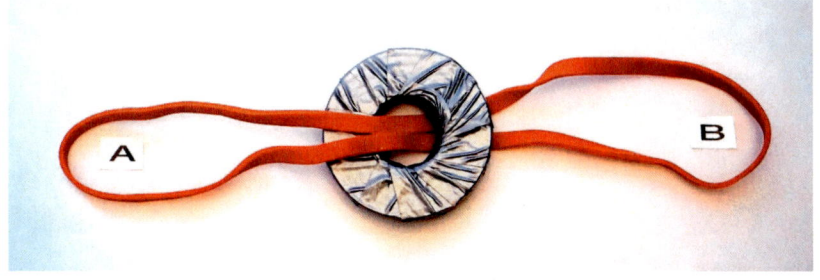

STEP 8 Then, take the other end (B) of the rubber band, and place it flat into the opening of the (A) loop.

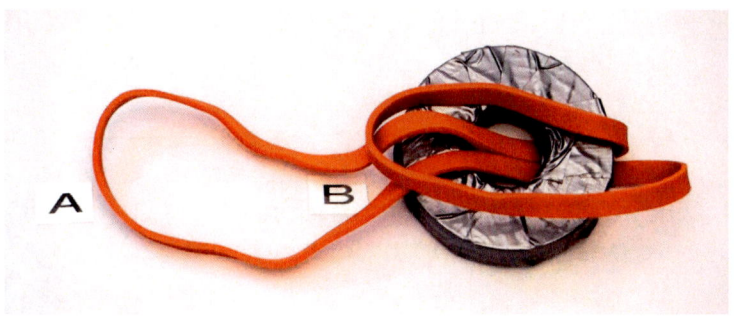

TAMING IDIOPATHIC TOE WALKING

6 Design & Fabrication of "Toe Tamers"

♦ Directions on How to Construct "Toe Tamers":

STEP 9 Hold down the covered washers on the flat surface with one hand, and **thread the (B) end to pull through the (A) end** to the side to form a half or slip knot. The weight will automatically flip when the (B) end is pulled through (A).

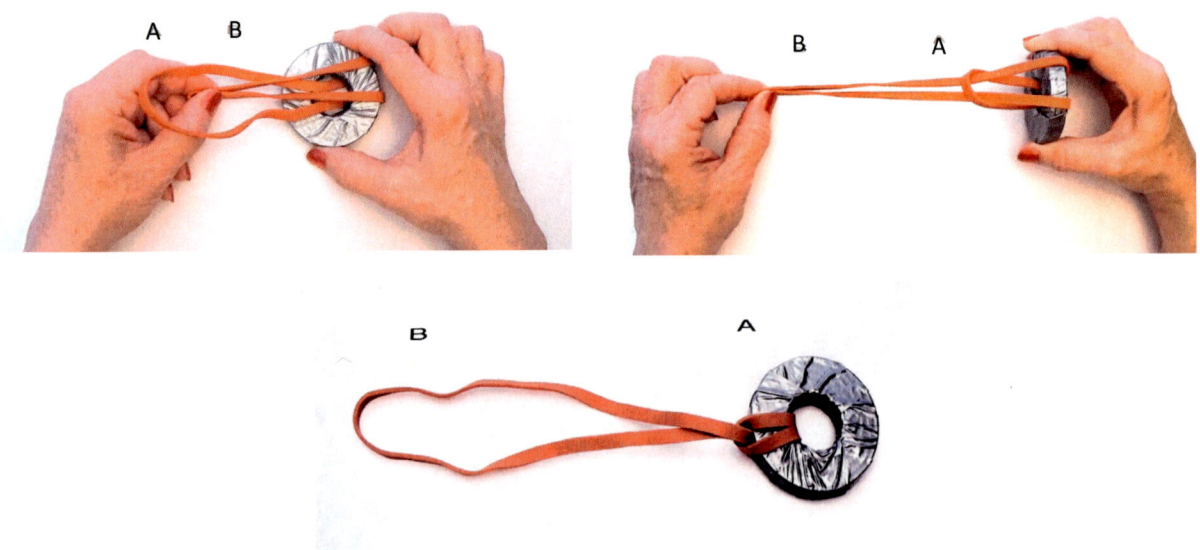

STEP 10 If a second rubber band is to be used for each shoe, then repeat step #7-9 on the opposite side of the opening of the "Toe Tamers" weights. It is generally advised to use the number of bands needed for optimum securement to be sure the weights do not move while walking.

NOTE OF CAUTION: "Toe Tamers" are not recommended for activities involving running, jumping, kicking, etc. due to the possibility of the weights detaching, becoming a projectile, and possibly hitting or injuring someone.

6 Design & Fabrication of "Toe Tamers"

♦ **Sample "Toe Tamer"*:**

Patterned duct tape selected by Carlie, one of the females in the case studies.

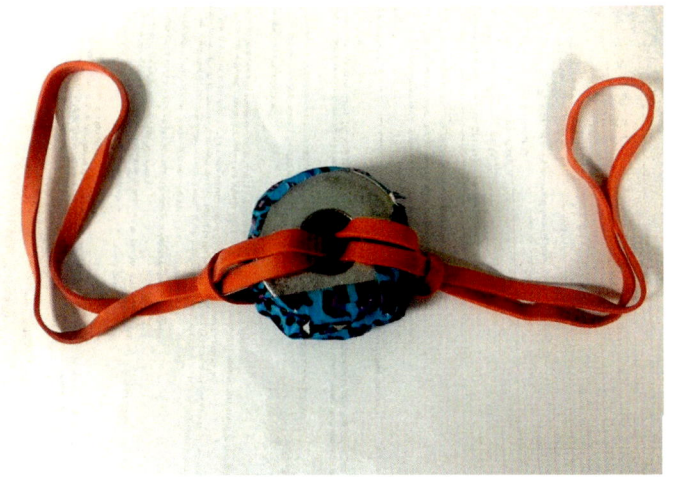
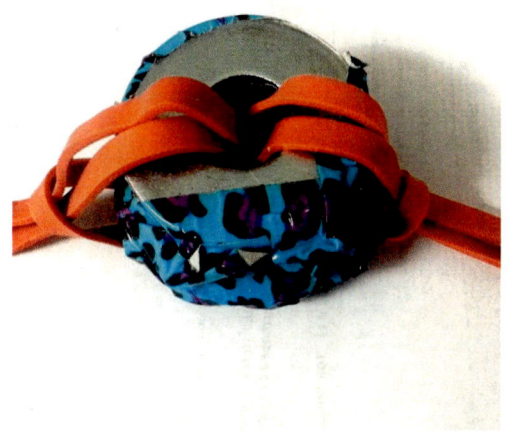
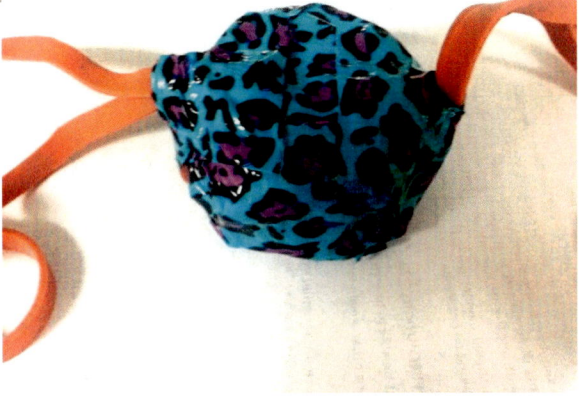
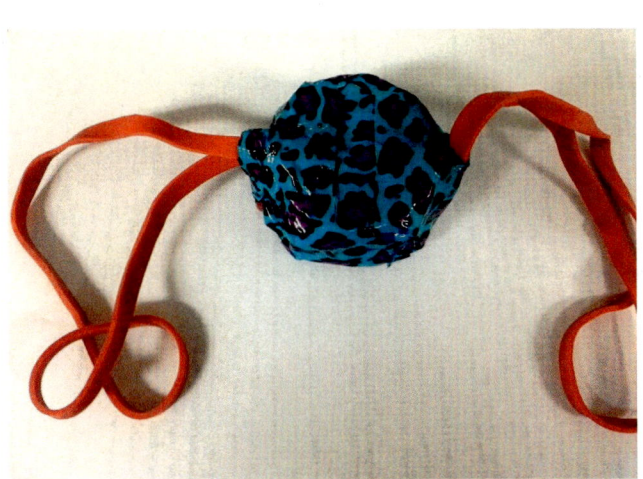

*Without Stabilizer

TAMING IDIOPATHIC TOE WALKING 21

6 Design & Fabrication of "Toe Tamers"

♦ <u>Sample "Toe Tamer"</u>*:

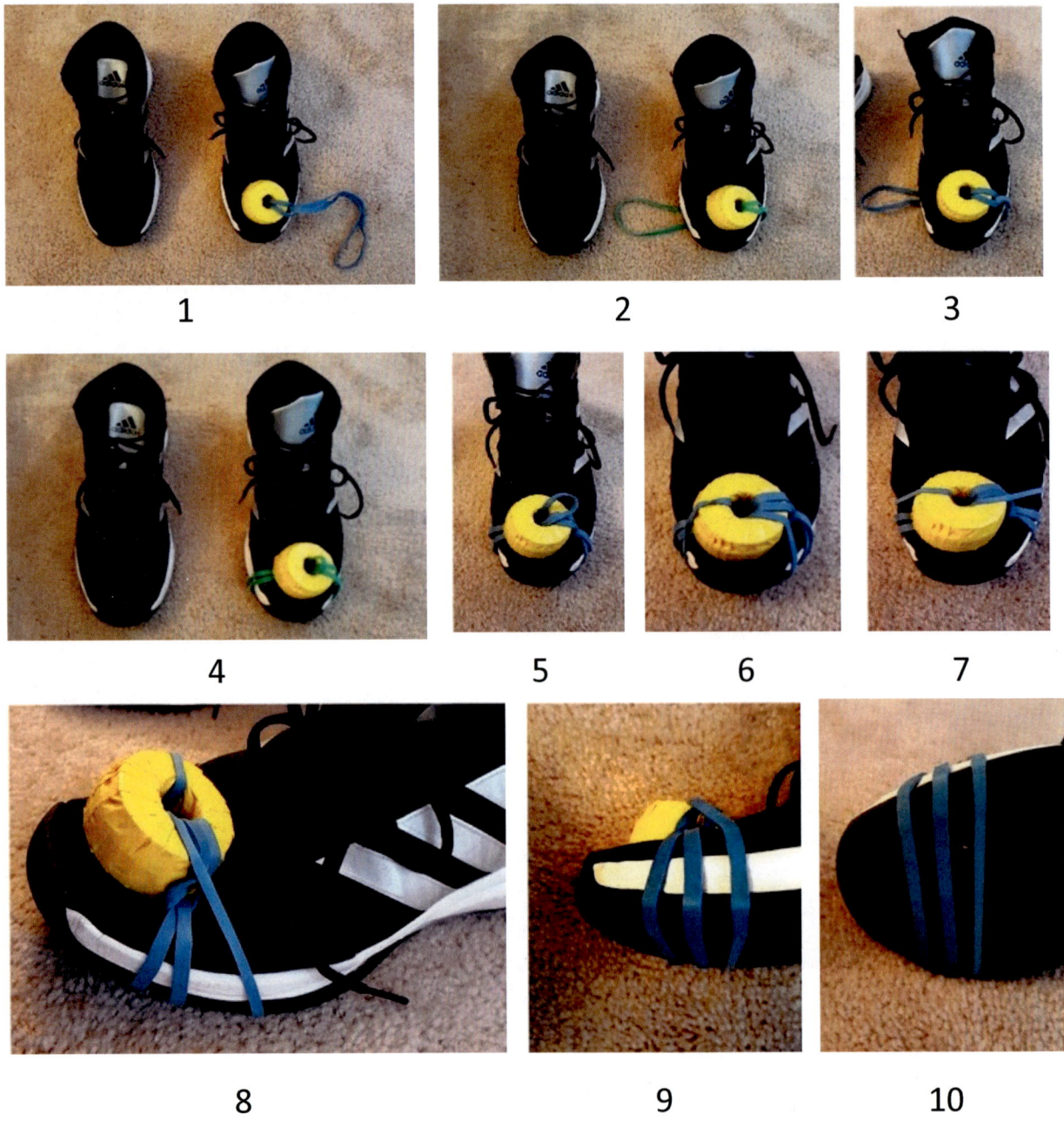

*Above images are without the addition of a stabilizer (ankle loop) band. When a stabilizer band is added, the foot would be inserted into the loop first before adding the Toe Tamer and its attached toe end band(s).

TAMING IDIOPATHIC TOE WALKING

6 Design & Fabrication of "Toe Tamers"

♦ Directions on How to Construct "Toe Tamers"

STEP 11 TO ADD A STABILIZER BAND: Loop an additional band inside the center ring of the Toe Tamer. Orient the weight so it is perpendicular to the other band(s) on the circular weight. This band can then be placed with both loops on top of each other for the child or person to insert the foot inside the double loop opening so the additional band wraps behind the ankle. This gives the Toe Tamer three points of contact for greater stability. It reduces the chances of the weights slipping off the shoe, and adds another step in case a child attempts to remove the weight.

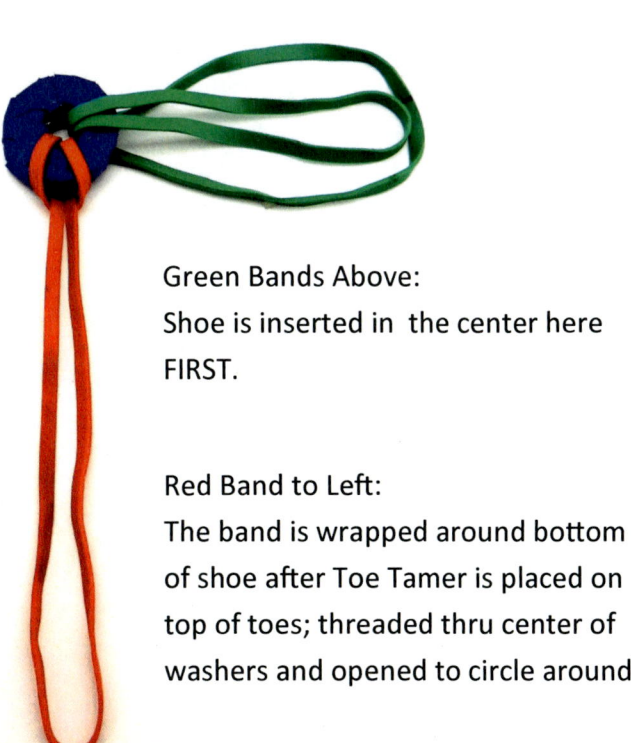

Green Bands Above:
Shoe is inserted in the center here FIRST.

Red Band to Left:
The band is wrapped around bottom of shoe after Toe Tamer is placed on top of toes; threaded thru center of washers and opened to circle around

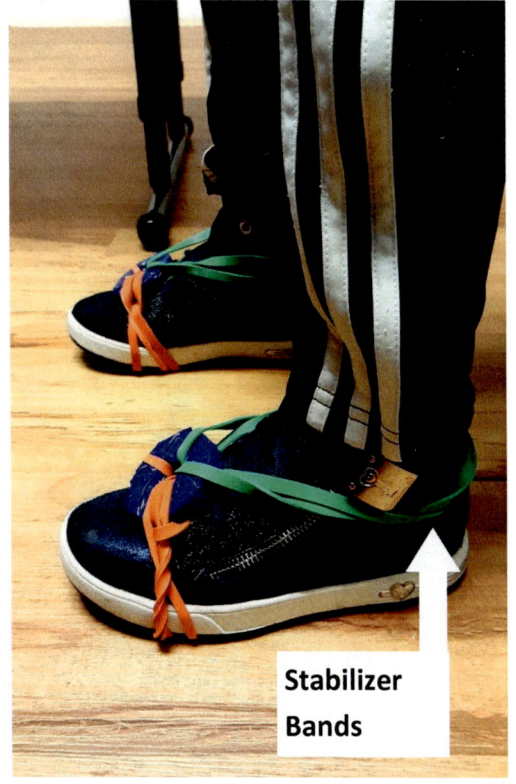

Stabilizer Bands

[Once the construction of the "Toe Tamers" has been completed, proceed to the section on How to Place the "Toe Tamers".]

TAMING IDIOPATHIC TOE WALKING

7 Protocol for Placing of "Toe Tamers"

◆ *Directions for Placing "Tamers":*

STEP 1 **Hold the "Toe Tamer" with the loops** coming out the top (if 1 band) or the sides (if 2 bands used) of the assembly.

STEP 2 **For 1 band used...**
   A. Place the weight on top of the shoe where the ball of the foot would be inside the shoe.

   B. Take the looped or "U" shaped band from the side to wrap under the shoe and around to the other side to return to the top of the shoe.

   C. Then, thread the end of the same loop (double bands) under and through the opening of the "Toe Tamer" to come out the top of the center opening.

   D. Open the band to wrap it completely around the end of the shoe once again to form a circle around the toes with a single band this time. This should produce a snug fit that will not allow the weight to move when walking.

STEP 3 **For 2 bands used...**
   A. Wrap each double band around the toe of the shoe.

   B. Then, open each band at the top of the shoe form a circle.

   C. Wrap each circle to go over the toe end to form a double wrap of bands. This should secure the "Toe Tamers" very snugly though a slight lift of the toe end may be noticeable. This should not interfere with the more typical gait pattern of heel strike to toe lift. It has been noticed to increase the amount of toe lifting that occurs which would further help the lengthening of the heel cords if they are already slightly shortened.

7 Protocol for Placing of "Toe Tamers"

♦ *Directions for Placing "Tamers":*

STEP 3 (Continued)-

> **NOTE:** If the heel cords are shortened significantly, the "Toe Tamers" may need to be gradually applied to build up tolerance, and allow the heel cords to naturally stretch with the heel moving closer to the floor with each use. The progress of this action can be seen by using a ruler next to the heel of each foot after the "Toe Tamer" has been re moved to measure the number of inches off the floor before the foot is completely down and resting flat on the floor.
>
> [See example in Section 9.]

STEP 4 Stability Bands [Recommended]

Use of stability bands are recommended to provide three points of contact to keep Toe Tamers securely in place for added stability. If use of these bands are desired...

A. Select a third band that is close to equal to the distance from the toes to the front of the ankle, preferably after attached through the inside of the washer weight.

B. Attach this additional band perpendicular to the toe bands through the center of the washers to form a "T" design. [It will lie on top along the midline of the shoe.]

C. Have the individual step into this band before the "Toe Tamers" are placed so that this adds as a third point of contact to stabilize the unit from slipping off the shoe.

8 Protocol for Wearing "Toe Tamers"

♦ *<u>Recommended Schedule for Use:</u>*

Suggested use of "Toe Tamers" will vary, depending on the age of the child and the severity of the toe walking behaviors. For young children ages 3-6 years of age, typical use times have been from 2-4 months for an average of 2-3 hours per day for 5-6 days per week.

For children 7 years and older that have consistently toe walked, the time could increase to 4-9 months for 3-4 hours daily.

AGE RANGE	HOURS PER DAY*	NO. OF MONTHS
3 to 6 YEARS OLD	2-3	2-4
7 YEARS & OLDER	3-4	4-9

*Based on usage rate of 5-6 days per week and dependent on degree or severity of toe walking.

Once the child no longer needs this input, s/he should be able to maintain a typical heel-toe walking pattern when bare footed. If not, continued use is recommended to help further integrate and maintain this desired gait or walking pattern.

The calming will be evident when the child can walk in a typical pattern with shoes on, but without the "Toe Tamers" in place. Then, the child will be able to maintain the feet on the floor once socks and shoes are removed. The child should continue the flat footed stance and no further toe walking once full integration or sensory saturation has been achieved.

TAMING IDIOPATHIC TOE WALKING

OCCUPATIONAL /PHYSICAL THERAPY
TOE WEIGHTS ["Toe Tamers"™] FORM

Note to therapists: Parents should be informed prior to regular use of toe weights in the classroom or clinic with a child. This form should be completed (following an initial trial of 1-2 weeks) if toe weights are to become part of a child's daily sensory strategy plan, especially if in the home and/or classroom. An exchange of feedback is recommended among the therapist, teacher and parent to occur following the first 2 weeks of a formal wearing schedule.

-Toe weights should be recommended/distributed by a therapist for a specific student for a specific reason. Toe weights must be correctly designed for effectiveness for each student. The child's weight will determine the amount of weights to be used per shoe/ foot.

-A wearing schedule for toe weights should be developed collaboratively. Use should be during periods of supervision to monitor positioning and safety.

-Toe weights should not be worn longer than 2–3 hours maximum at one time, depending on the child's age. Wearing tolerance and endurance should be gradually increased from increments of 30 minutes to prevent over stretching of the calf muscles which could cause discomfort. If full range of motion is present, and the use is preventative in nature, then use may be up to 3-4 hours, as tolerated.

-The therapist should monitor the use of the toe weights and the wearing schedule as needed, determining the baseline wearing time based on observations of the child's initial tolerance of the shoes with the weights.

REMINDERS / PRECAUTIONS:

-The child must be able to tolerate the toe weights for at least 30 minutes duration.

-Toe weights must be discontinued if the child removes them immediately and/or uses them as a toy or projectile.

-Toe weights or other weighted items should not be used as a punishment or to reinforce undesirable behavior.

Toe weights are not recommended for children with significantly atypical neuromuscular status, spinal malalignment, weakened respiratory status and/or generalized weakness. The basis for the toe walking must be idiopathic or of unknown origin, not orthopedic or neurological, in nature, for this sensory strategy to be appropriate and effective.

Child: _____ **School:** _____ **Weight of each "Toe Tamer":** _____ ozs.

Purpose:

_____ To reduce toe walking and facilitate a more normal heel-toe gait pattern.

_____ To stretch and lengthen the calf muscles/tendons, and enable child to stand flat footed.

_____ To improve tolerance for wearing ☐ socks ☐ shoes.

_____ Other:_____

Recommended schedule of use (List specific activities and/or times as needed):

_____ 30 minutes on/ 30 minutes off for _____ period of time _____

_____ 60 minutes on/ 30 minutes off for _____ period of time _____

_____ 90 minutes on/ 30 minutes off for _____ period of time _____

_____ 2.0 hours on/ 30 minutes off during the week day except during: _____

_____ Other time specific wearing schedule:_____

Therapist:_____ Date:_____

Parent:_____ Date:_____

Teacher/Caregiver: _____ Date:_____

ISM/© 2017

TERAPIA OCUPACIONAL O FÍSICA
PLANILLA PARA PESAS DE LOS DEDOS DE LOS PIES ["Toe Tamers"™]

Nota para los terapistas: Los padres deben de ser informados antes del uso regular de las pesas de los dedos de los pies en la clase o en la clínica con el niño. Esta forma debe ser completada (siguiente 1-2 semanas de prueba inicial) si las pesas de los dedos de los pies van a ser parte de la rutina diaria del niño como la estrategia sensorial, especialmente, si se usan en la casa o la clase. Es recomendado el intercambio verbal entre el/ la terapista, la maestra, y los padres después de las primeras 2 semanas del programa cuando el niño haya caminado con las pesas siguiendo el régimen exacto del plan.

-Las pesas para los dedos de los pies deben ser recomendadas /distribuidas por un terapista específicamente para el alumno designado y por la razón específica. Las pesas para los dedos de los pies deben de ser diseñadas correctamente para la eficacia de cada estudiante. El peso del niño determinará la cantidad de pesas que se usaran para cada zapato/pie.

-Un programa para el uso de las peas de los dedos de los pies debe ser desarrollado colaborativamente bajo supervisión y por el período de tiempo especificado, para monitorear la posición de las pesas y la seguridad del niño.

-Las pesas de los dedos de los pies no se deben usar por más de 2-3 horas máximas cada vez, dependiendo de la edad del niño. La tolerancia del uso de las pesas y la resistencia del uso vendrá gradualmente al añadir más tiempo cada vez en incrementos de 30 minutos para prevenir que los músculos de la pantorrilla sean muy estrechados, causando así incomodidad. Si el niño tiene rango completo de movimiento y si el uso es mayormente preventivo, entonces el uso de las pesas puede ser de 3-4 horas, según sean toleradas.

-El terapista debe monitorear el uso de las pesas de los dedos de los pies y el régimen dictado para ellas como sea necesario, determinando la línea de base establecida para el uso de las pesas basada en observar la tolerancia inicial del niño usando las pesas en los zapatos.

RECORDATORIO / PRECAUCIONES:

-El niño tiene que ser capaz de tolerar el peso de las pesas por lo menos 30 minutos de duración continua.

-Las pesas deben ser descontinuadas si el niño se las quita inmediatamente o las usa como un juguete o proyectil.

-Estas pesas o cualquier pesa no se debe usar como castigo o para reforzar el comportamiento indeseable del niño.

Las pesas de los dedos de los pies no son recomendadas para los niños con significante estado anormal neuromuscular, o desalineación de la columna vertebral, estado respiratorio débil y/o debilidad general. La causa del caminar en las puntas de los pies debe ser idiopático o por causa desconocida no por causa ortopédica o neurológica, para que esta estrategia sensorial sea apropiada y efectiva.

Nombre del niño:_____ Escuela:_____ Peso de cada "Toe Tamer": _____ozs.

Propósito:

_____ Para reducir el caminar en los dedos de los pies y facilitar la pisada normal desde el talón hasta las puntas de los pies.

_____ Para estrechar los músculos de la pantorrilla/ tendones, y permitir que el niño pueda pararse con los pies planos.

_____ Para mejorar la tolerancia de calzar o usar ☐calcetines (medias) ☐ zapatos.

_____ Otro:_____

Recomendaciones para el uso por el tiempo especificado (especifique las actividades y/o el tiempo, como sea necesario):

_____ 30 minutos de práctica/ 30 minutes sin práctica para _____período de tiempo _____

_____ 60 minutos de práctica/ 30 minutos sin práctica para _____ período de tiempo _____

_____ 90 minutos de práctica / 30 minutos sin práctica para _____período de tiempo_____

_____ 2.0 minutos de práctica/30 minutos sin práctica durante la semana excepto cuando: _____

_____ Itinerario para usarlo en cualquier otro tiempo:_____

Terapista:_____ Fecha:_____

Padre o Madre:_____ Fecha:_____

Maestra(o)/Cuidador(a): _____ Fecha:_____

9 Wearing Record (Sample)

Name: **Joey Ontoesies** Age: **7-9 years**
Purpose of "Toe Tamers": **Calm toes to keep on socks & shoes**

DATE	TIME WORN [Hours]	PROGRESS *
11-02-15	2.5	First fitting of "Toe Tamers" [TT]; tolerated 2.5 hours well before asked to remove. Heels were each measured at 3.75" off the floor. ISM
11-03-15	3.0	Increased tolerance for TT without complaints; no change in heel ht. ISM
11-04-15	3.25	Increased tolerance w/o complaints; heels now 3.5" off floor. ISM
11-05-15	3.5	Tolerance increased w/o complaints; heels now 3.0" off floor. ISM

ISM/©2017   [* Note Example: Number of inches the heel(s) is/are off the floor.]

TAMING IDIOPATHIC TOE WALKING

9 Wearing Record

Name of Child: _____ Age: _____ years

Purpose of "Toe Tamers": _____

DATE	TIME WORN [Hours]	PROGRESS *

[* Note Example: Number of inches the heel(s) is/are off the floor.]

9 Wearing Graph

Name of Child: _____   Age: _____ years

Purpose of "Toe Tamers": _____

Recorder: _____ Period Tracked: _____ to _____

Progress Record for Reducing Toe Walking										
Dates										
Measure in Inches of Heel Center from Floor/Flat Surface	Inches 6.0									
	5.5									
	5.0									
	4.5									
	4.0									
	3.5									
	3.0									
	2.5									
	2.0									
	1.5									
	1.0									
	.50									
	Flat									

ISM/©2017   [NOTE: Graph should show descending line when progressing to reduce heel height off floor.]

ISM/©2017

TAMING IDIOPATHIC TOE WALKING

9 Wearing Record

Name of Child: _____ Age: _____ years

Purpose of "Toe Tamers": _____

DATE	TIME WORN [Hours]	PROGRESS *

ISM/©2017 [* Note Example: Number of inches the heel(s) is/are off the floor.]

9 Wearing Graph

Name of Child: _____   Age: _____ years

Purpose of "Toe Tamers": _____

Recorder: _____ Period Tracked: _____ to _____

Progress Record for Reducing Toe Walking

Dates										
Inches 6.0										
5.5										
5.0										
4.5										
4.0										
3.5										
3.0										
2.5										
2.0										
1.5										
1.0										
.50										
Flat										

Measure in Inches of Heel Center from Floor/Flat Surface

ISM/©2017   [NOTE: Graph should show descending line when progressing to reduce heel height off floor.]

ISM/©2017

TAMING IDIOPATHIC TOE WALKING   35

9 Wearing Record

Name of Child: _____ Age: _____ years

Purpose of "Toe Tamers": _____

DATE	TIME WORN [Hours]	PROGRESS *

ISM/©2017   [* Note Example: Number of inches the heel(s) is/are off the floor.]

9 Wearing Graph

Name of Child: _____ Age: _____ years

Purpose of "Toe Tamers": _____

Recorder: _____ Period Tracked: _____ to _____

	Progress Record for Reducing Toe Walking								
Dates									
Measure in Inches of Heel Center from Floor/Flat Surface	Inches 6.0								
	5.5								
	5.0								
	4.5								
	4.0								
	3.5								
	3.0								
	2.5								
	2.0								
	1.5								
	1.0								
	.50								
	Flat								

ISM/©2017   [NOTE: Graph should show descending line when progressing to reduce heel height off floor.]

ISM/©2017

TAMING IDIOPATHIC TOE WALKING

9 Wearing Record

Name of Child: _____ Age: _____ years

Purpose of "Toe Tamers": _____

DATE	TIME WORN [Hours]	PROGRESS *

[* Note Example: Number of inches the heel(s) is/are off the floor.]

9 Wearing Graph

Name of Child: _____ Age: _____ years

Purpose of "Toe Tamers": _____

Recorder: _____ Period Tracked: _____ to _____

Progress Record for Reducing Toe Walking								
Dates								
Measure in Inches of Heel Center from Floor/Flat Surface	Inches							
	6.0							
	5.5							
	5.0							
	4.5							
	4.0							
	3.5							
	3.0							
	2.5							
	2.0							
	1.5							
	1.0							
	.50							
	Flat							

ISM/©2017   [NOTE: Graph should show descending line when progressing to reduce heel height off floor.]

ISM/©2017

TAMING IDIOPATHIC TOE WALKING

9 Wearing Record

Name of Child: _____ Age: _____ years

Purpose of "Toe Tamers": _____

DATE	TIME WORN [Hours]	PROGRESS *

ISM/©2017 [* Note Example: Number of inches the heel(s) is/are off the floor.]

9 Wearing Graph

Name of Child: _____ Age: _____ years

Purpose of "Toe Tamers": _____

Recorder: _____ Period Tracked: _____ to _____

Progress Record for Reducing Toe Walking										
Dates										
Measure in Inches of Heel Center from Floor/Flat Surface	Inches 6.0									
	5.5									
	5.0									
	4.5									
	4.0									
	3.5									
	3.0									
	2.5									
	2.0									
	1.5									
	1.0									
	.50									
	Flat									

ISM/©2017   [NOTE: Graph should show descending line when progressing to reduce heel height off floor.]

10 Case Studies

◆ Camden...
6 year old male child with severe Sensory Processing Disorder [SPD]:

Camden was in the first grade, and had walked on his toes since he began bearing weight on his feet. His toe walking was so extreme that he would not keep his socks and shoes on his feet in the classroom or in the home. When he got excited, he would not only walk on the tips of his toes, but he would then bend or flex the end joint of his toes, and walk on the *back* of his toes which appeared painful to those that watched him do so! He appeared to have a high pain tolerance level based on this pattern of stance.

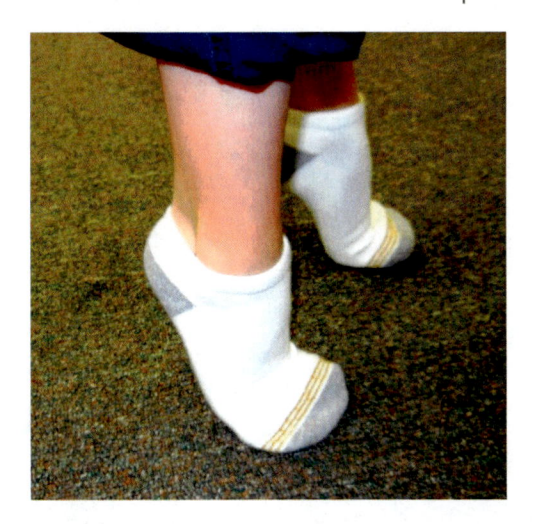

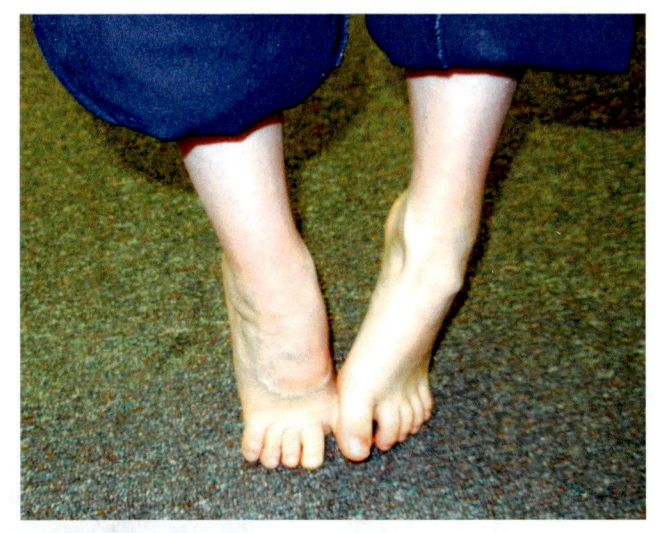

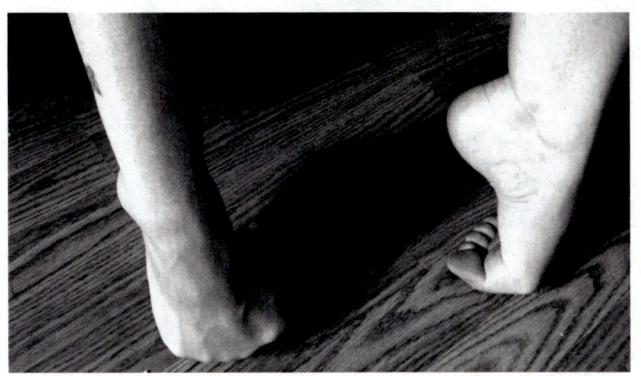

Without his socks and shoes, Camden weighed 64 pounds. When this weight was divided by 10, the amount determined to be needed was 6.5 ounces of weights for each "Toe Tamer". This weight was rounded down to 6 ounces for fabrication of the "Toe Tamers".

TAMING IDIOPATHIC TOE WALKING

10 Case Studies

♦ Camden...
6 year old male child with severe Sensory Processing Disorder [SPD]:

Once the "Toe Tamers' were placed on Camden's shoes, he was able to complete a typical heel-toe gait or walking pattern. Camden actually lifted the toe of his shoe before lifting his heel to place and step forward to walk with his heels on the floor or ground. He also kept his shoes and socks on his feet while in the classroom and throughout the school when they were used. When Camden walked down the halls or into the lunchroom, school staff noticed his ability to walk with his feet down, and often made favorable remarks to his teacher.

Camden's teacher was instructed on the use protocol, and a copy was sent home for the parents' signatures for use in school. The use of the "Toe Tamers' were also recommended for use in the home in the evenings as tolerated, as well as on the weekends to continue the sensory input on a consistent basis throughout the week. This would further help Camden to satiate the need his body apparently had for pressure or proprioceptive input into the balls of the feet to "calm" his heel lift or atypical toe walking behaviors.

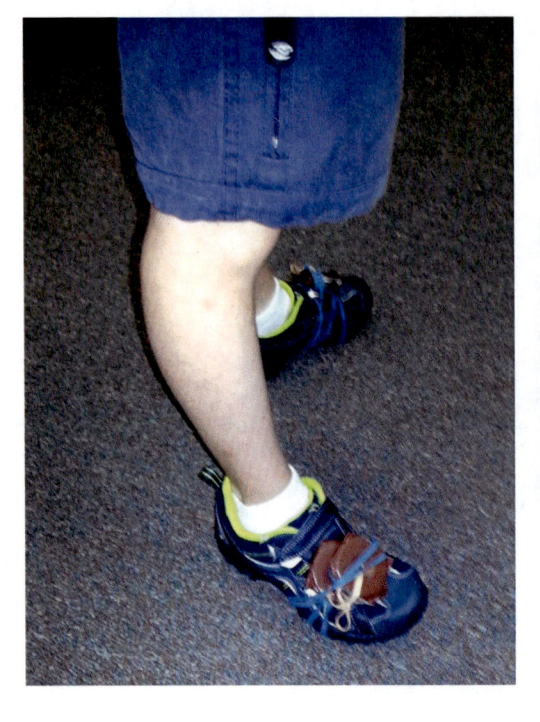

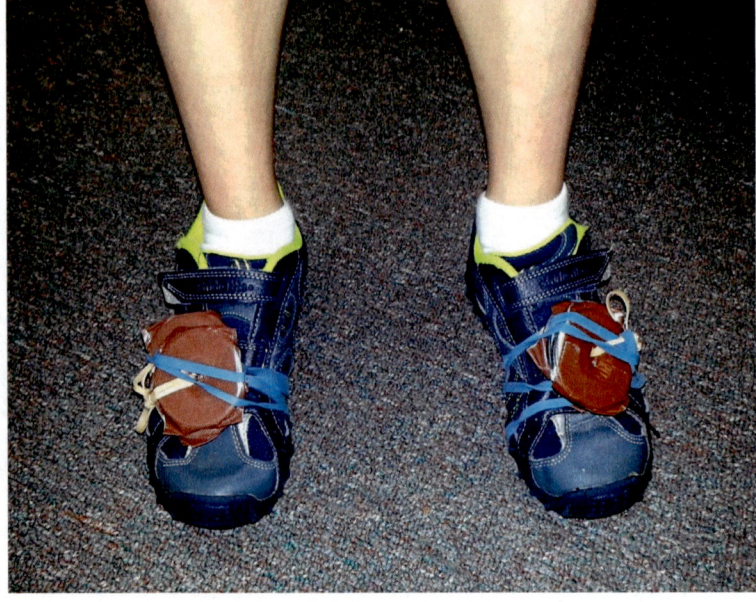

TAMING IDIOPATHIC TOE WALKING

10 Case Studies

♦ Carlie…
15 year old female adolescent with severe Autism Spectrum Disorder [ASD]:

Carlie was in a combined, self-contained, Special Education class at the middle school level for children with severe Autism and Intellectual Disabilities. This meant that close supervision for the use of the Toe Tamers could be provided.

On first observation Carlie was seen wearing AFO's or Ankle Foot Orthoses which are splints to hold the ankles at 90 degree angles. This limited movement of each foot and ankle as a unit. When the teacher was asked why she was wearing the ankle braces with orthopedic type shoes with Velcro closures, the reason given was simply due to her severe toe walking behaviors. The basis of the toe walking was further questioned, and there was reportedly no underlying, identified orthopedic or neurological problem. This was verified by the school Physical Therapist upon consultation with this Occupational Therapist.

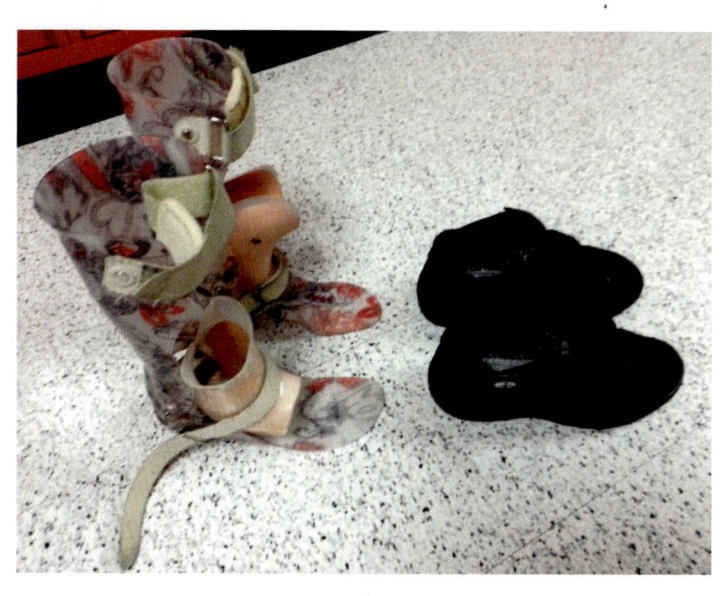

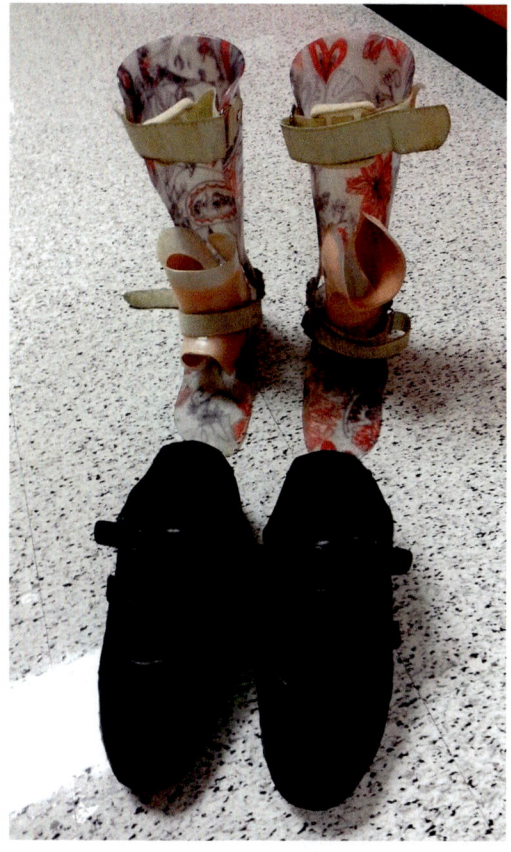

TAMING IDIOPATHIC TOE WALKING

10 Case Studies

♦ Carlie…
15 year old female adolescent with severe Autism Spectrum Disorder [ASD]:

A note was then sent home to the parents to ask if they would be interested in trying an alternative treatment technique to enable Carlie to wear typical teenage tennis shoes on which a pair of "Toe Tamers" would be added to help remedy her toe walking behavior. The parents gave the teacher permission to proceed that was relayed to this O.T. The teacher had Carlie weighed, and a weight of 143 pounds was recorded and reported to this therapist.

Carlie's total body weight was divided by 10. This yielded a rounded measure of 14 ounces for the maximum amount of weight to be added to each shoe's "Toe Tamer".

A combination of 1.0 to 2.5 ounce weights were then used to get a total weight equal to 14.0 ounces per "Toe Tamer". The weights were secured by the use of two, sturdy 14 inch rubber bands with a brightly patterned pink, turquoise and black leopard printed duct tape that was chosen by Carlie. It was very color coordinated with the hot, pink, laced tennis shoes that were sent in by her parents for this sensory strategy application.

Carlie's braces were removed to change her shoes. This therapist noted that her toes were so tightly pointed that they were in a straight line with her leg! It was not clear if this strategy Would be effective enough to override this extreme ankle to toe position.

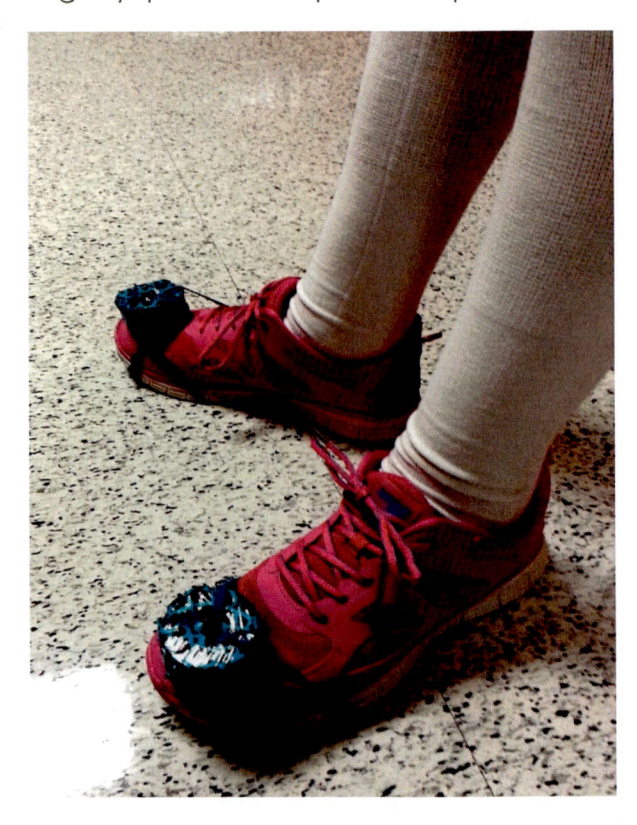

TAMING IDIOPATHIC TOE WALKING

10 Case Studies

♦ Carlie...
15 year old female adolescent with severe Autism Spectrum Disorder [ASD]:

The "Toe Tamers" were then placed on her shoes while she sat at her desk. They were secured on the top of the brightly colored tennis shoes that appeared very typical for a teenage girl this age.

On Carlie's initial stance, she looked down at her feet, and she did not move. She required prompting to walk from her desk to the door and down the hallway for a distance of approximately 30 feet. When she did, she immediately placed her heels down on the floor and lifted the toe of each foot before placing the next foot forward in a typical gait pattern for walking. Though she continued with a rotated hip pattern where her feet turned outward, the pattern exhibited from her heel to her toe were much like the typical pattern used by any other teen to walk.

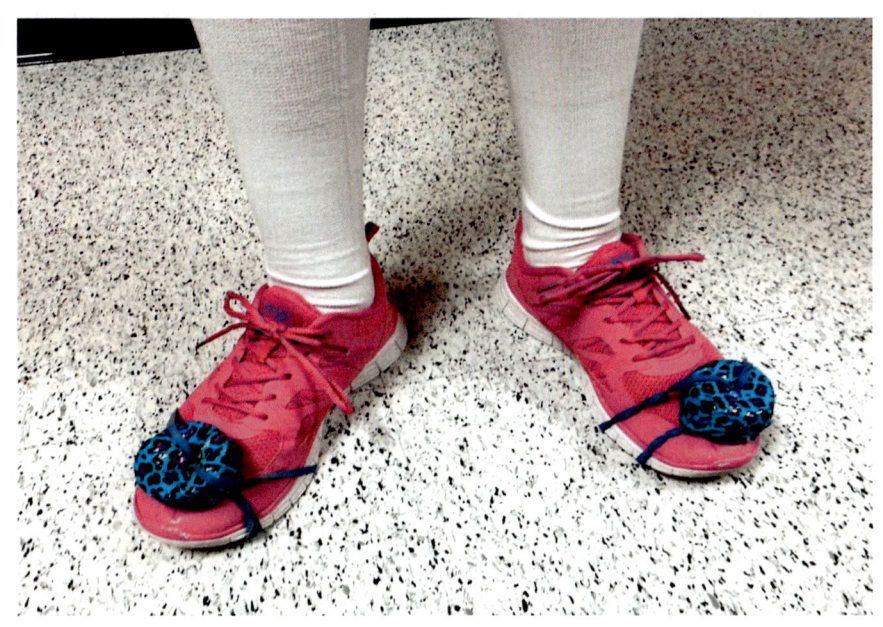

NOTE OF CAUTION: *Due to the severity of her disability, the use of these "Toe Tamers" needed to be supervised to ensure appropriate usage. They were not worn outside of Carlie's classroom until usage became more routine to insure that she would not remove them or that they would not slip off during extended periods of walking. These weights could be misused if they were found by peers that did not know their intended use. Also, "Toe Tamers" should only be used when walking in a standing/upright position to provide the optimum proprioceptive input that is needed to calm or inhibit plantar flexion and relax the toes.*

TAMING IDIOPATHIC TOE WALKING

10 Case Studies

◆ Carlie...
15 year old female adolescent with severe Autism Spectrum Disorder [ASD]:

Carlie's vocabulary was limited; however, she could express thoughts in short phrases. Once she began walking with the Toe Tamers, she was asked, "How do they feel?" Her reply, "A lot heavier!" She was then asked if that was good or bad. She then replied, "Heavier good!" She pointed to her right foot and indicated, "[It] wants to get on toes a little bit." Then, she pointed to her left foot, and added, "Nope. It does not want to [get on toes]."

When Carlie was asked if the Toe Tamers were easy or hard to wear, she stated they were, "Easy", but then added that they, "Hurt my leg a little bit." She then grabbed the back of her thigh and calf, possibly due to the feeling of being stretched. At this point she had been walking with the Toe Tamers for a total of approximately 2 hours that morning.

When the Toe Tamers were removed after wearing them for a total of 3 hours in the morning at school, Carlie remarked, "Still feels like its on my shoe when it's off!" The proprioceptive input lingered even after removal. The skin on her feet and toes were checked daily, and no pressure lines or skin breakdowns were ever reported or noticed.

Though the Toe Tamers were sent home for use over the summer break, their continued use was not known. Carlie was scheduled to return to this class in the Fall; however, this therapist did not return to work in this county school system. Carlie's teacher also transferred to work in another school, so this therapist could not monitor progress through her either. These are factors to consider when recommending and implementing the use of therapeutic equipment provided to the parent for use over summer breaks, especially if monitoring by either OT or PT will not be provided through Extended School Year or ESY services.

10 Case Studies

◆ Vanessa...
6 year old female with moderate Autism Spectrum Disorder [ASD]:

Vanessa would regularly scream, bite and run whenever attempts were made to engage her in activities in the clinic or at school, especially if she was asked to remove her shoes and socks. She was overly sensitive tactually, and would scream, "Ouch!" whenever any part of her body was lightly touched or accidentally brushed. To engage her to walk to the clinic, "active grasp" was used by saying, "Hold my finger" instead of grasping her hand. This way she controlled the input and it was possible for this therapist to "feel" when she was preparing to run. In summary, Vanessa demonstrated tactile defensiveness or aversiveness and was in constant "flight" mode with poor self-regulation or self-calming abilities.

Additionally, Vanessa was so hyperactive and restless that it was not possible to take a clear, still photo of her with her shoes donned before use of her Toe Tamers. Her toe walking was most evident with use of her sandals, but even with her tennis shoes, she would walk with approximately 2-2.5 inches off the floor consistently.

Vanessa's mother agreed to use of the Toe Tamers at home on a daily basis, as much as she would tolerate them. Surprisingly, when the Toe Tamers were made, she displayed an interest in them. She also allowed her mother and this O.T. to place them on her shoes without any screaming or fighting. She immediately responded to the proprioceptive input by walking with her feet flat on the floor for at least 6 of 10 steps taken.
Because of her initial hyperactivity, the use of stabilizers was added to prevent slippage or ease of removal by her.

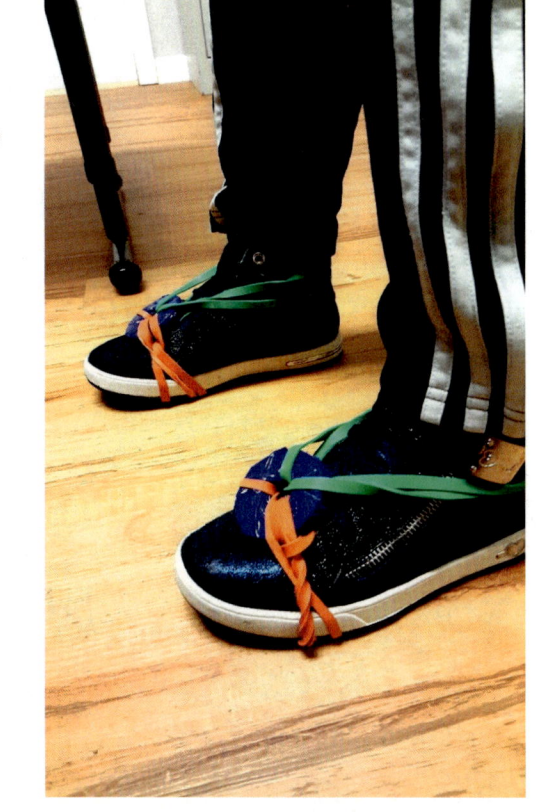

TAMING IDIOPATHIC TOE WALKING

10 Case Studies

♦ Vanessa…
6 year old female with moderate Autism Spectrum Disorder [ASD]:

Vanessa made no efforts to remove the Toe Tamers in the clinic when they were initially placed after the final weight and band adjustments. Per parent report, the Toe Tamers were used at home for up to three hours per day for 5 of 7 consecutive days of each of the first 3 weeks. Typically, she would have them placed on her shoes on arriving from school during the work week, and on weekends, would have them in place during the afternoons. She would have a break for two days per week before reapplying them again.

Vanessa's mother reported that she began walking flat footed within the second week of wearing the Toe Tamers. She returned the Toe Tamers after three months of consistent usage. Vanessa has continued to walk flat footed at home and in the clinic both with or without shoes during weekly visits four months after initial usage of the Toe Tamers. Her next short term objective is to remove her socks, and walk barefooted in the clinic. At home she will reportedly remove her own socks, and walks flat-footed without them, as well.

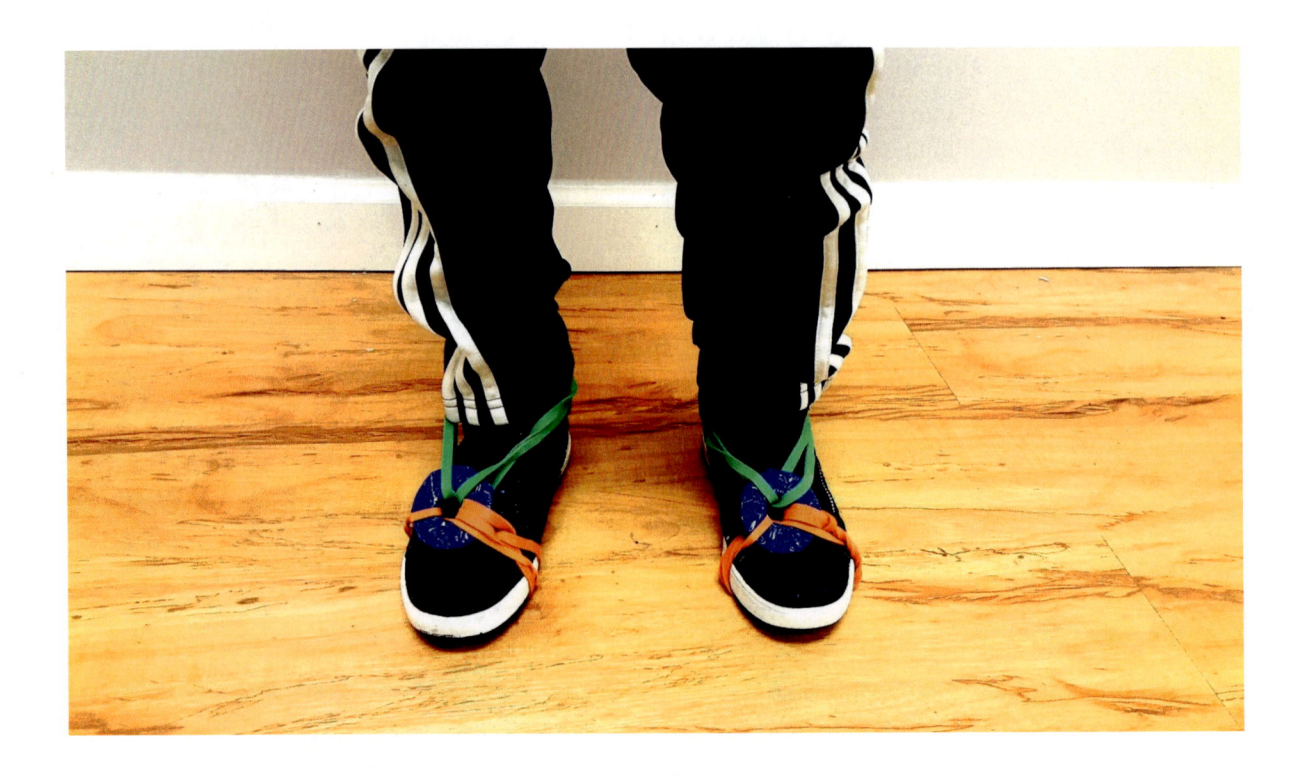

10 Case Studies

♦ Vanessa...
6 year old female with moderate Autism Spectrum Disorder [ASD]:

The photos below were taken after wearing Toe Tamers for two months. Vanessa's response was not typical of all children. Often it takes longer for a positive impact that is lasting; however, in Vanessa's case, three months after beginning usage, she no longer ran when asked to remove her shoes, and would independently remove them when asked. She still struggles to remove her socks in the clinic or to allow someone else to remove them other than her mother.

Since beginning use of her Toe Tamers, her participation and response to calming strategies improved significantly. She displays greater cooperation and focused attention to tasks both at home and during her clinic visits.

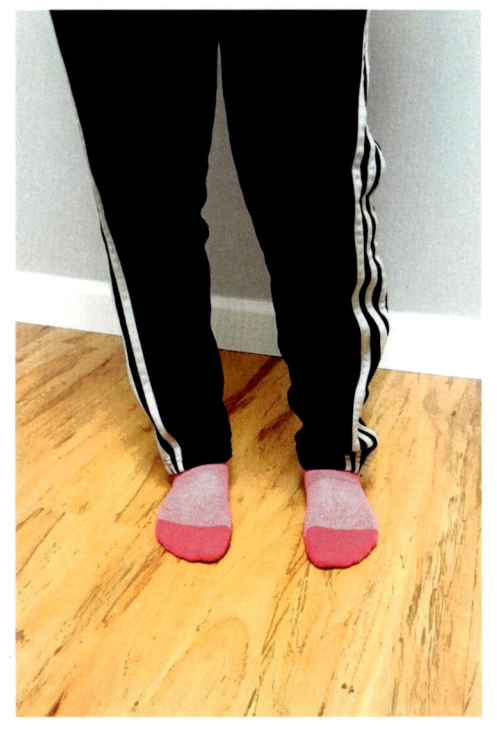

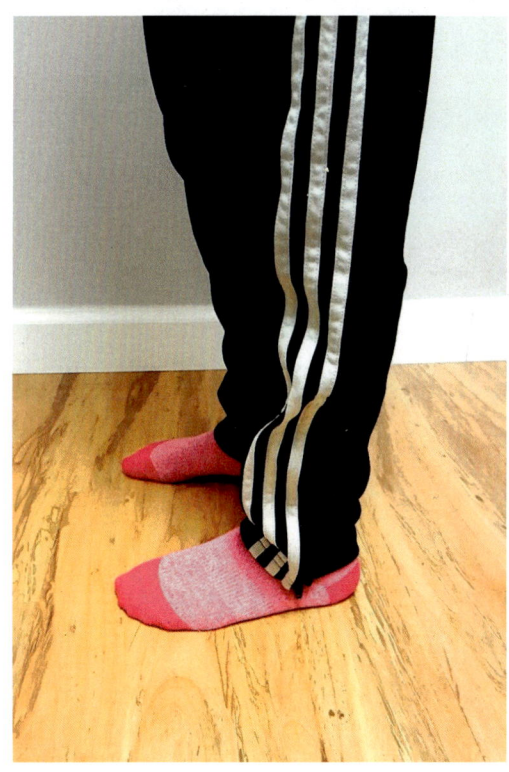

TAMING IDIOPATHIC TOE WALKING

11 References

WEBSITES:

- Toe Walking in Children; Brian Hoppestad, PT, MS, EdD; December 11, 2013; Vol. 24, Issue 22, page 16, Archives of Advance Healthcare Network for Physical Therapy and Rehab Medicine; *http://physical-therapy.advanceweb.com/Archives/Article-Archives/Toe-Walking-in-Children.asp*

- Toe Walking in Children: Definition; Mayo Clinic Staff; August 27, 2014; pp. 1; Mayo Clinic; *http://www.mayoclinic.org/diseases-conditions/toe-walking/basics/definition/con-20034585*

- Toe Walking in Children: Causes; Mayo Clinic Staff; August 27, 2014; pp. 1; Mayo Clinic; *http://www.mayoclinic.org/diseases-conditions/toe-walking/basics/causes/con-20034585*

- Toe Walking in Children: Symptoms; Mayo Clinic Staff; August 27, 2014; pp. 1; Mayo Clinic; *http://www.mayoclinic.org/diseases-conditions/toe-walking/basics/symptoms/con-20034585*

- Toe Walking in Children: Risk Factors; Mayo Clinic Staff; August 27, 2014; pp. 1; Mayo Clinic; *http://www.mayoclinic.org/diseases-conditions/toe-walking/basics/risk-factors/con-20034585*

- Toe Walking in Children: Complications; Mayo Clinic Staff; August 27, 2014; pp. 1; Mayo Clinic; *http://www.mayoclinic.org/diseases-conditions/toe-walking/basics/complications/con-20034585*

- Toe Walking in Children: Tests and Diagnosis; Mayo Clinic Staff; August 27, 2014; pp. 1; Mayo Clinic; *http://www.mayoclinic.org/diseases-conditions/toe-walking/basics/tests-diagnosis/con-20034585*

- Toe Walking in Children: Treatments and Drugs; Mayo Clinic Staff; August 27, 2014; pp. 1; Mayo Clinic; *http://www.mayoclinic.org/diseases-conditions/toe-walking/basics/treatment/con-20034585*

- Toe Walking: Symptoms & Behavior; Stephen M Edelson, Ph.D.; 2014; Autism Research Institute; *http://www.Globalautismcollaboration.com*

- Idiopathic Toe Walking: To Treat or not to Treat, that is the Question; Fred Dietz, MD and Songsak, Khunsree, MD; 2012; pp. 184-188; The IOWA Orthopaedic Journal; *http://www.ncbi.nim.nih.gov/pmc/articles/PMC3565400/*

- Toe Walking: Treatment & Management; Ryan Krochak, MD; Mark C Lee, MD; John S Early, MD; Francisco Talavera, PharmD, PhD; Dinesh Patel, MD, FACS; John H Calhoun, MD, FACS; Edwards P Schwentker, MD.; June 20, 2014; Medscape REFERENCE; *http://emedicine.medscape.com/article/1235248-treatment*

11 References

WEBSITES:

- Tips for Toe Walking; Lindsey Biel, OTR/L; July 17, 2013; Montana Autism Education Project (ddoty@mt.gov); *http://opi.mt.gov/users/dougdoty/weblog/3e778/Tips_for_Toe_Walking.html*

- Idiopathic Toe Walking; Area Education Agency 267 Special Education; September 14, 2014; Iowa; *http:// www.aea267.k12.ia.us/sped/services/physical-therapy/resources-for-parents-and-caregivers/toe-walking/*

- Children's Hospitals and Clinics of Minnesota Toe Walking Brochure: *https://www.aea267.k12.ia.us/?ACT=26&fid=5&d=1771&f=toe_walking_childrens_hospital_of_minnesota.pdf*

- Blank Children's Hospital Toe Walking Brochure: *https://www.aea267.k12.ia.us/system/assets/uploads/files/1771/toewalking-brochure-blank.pdf*

OTHER RESOURCES:

- Is Idiopathic Toe Walking Really Idiopathic? The motor skills and sensory processing abilities associated with idiopathic toe walking gait. Journal of Child Neurology, January, 2014; 29(1): 71-8. [Medline]

- Idiopathic Toe Talking and Sensory Processing Dysfunction; Cylie M Williams, Paul Tinley, and Michael Curtin; Journal of Foot Ankle Res.; August 16, 2010; 3:16; doi: 10.11861757-1146-3-16

- WASHERS: Everbilt flat washers distributed by Home Depot, Inc.
  The Fastener Center flat washers; Hillman Fastener, Cincinnati, Ohio 45231

- BANDS: SUPERSIZE BANDS: Oversized Bands for Big Jobs; Alliance Rubber Company, ©2013; Hot Springs, AR 71901; www.RUBBERBAND.com

- SCALE: Kamenstein by Lifetime Brands, Inc.; Corporate Headquarters-1000 Stewart Avenue, Garden City, NY 11530; questions@lifetimebrands.com; (516) 683-6000

- PHOTOGRAPHY: Case studies-actual former and current students and clinic patients of Ileana S. McCaigue, OTR/L; R.J. McCaigue; blog.dinopt.comfreephoto.png; free photo from baystatept.com; bubalu daycare center image from freephotos.jpg; pediatricsconsult-e60.comfreephotos.png; Bing free images

Ileana S. McCaigue, OTR/L

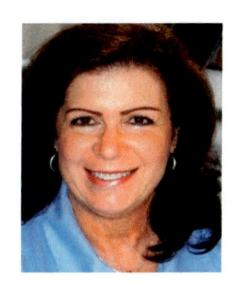

A 1977 summa cum laude graduate from the Medical College of Georgia in Augusta, Georgia, Ileana is an Occupational Therapist with 40 years of experience in the field of Occupational Therapy. She is nationally board certified/registered and licensed by the state of Georgia. She has specialty certifications in Sensory Integration, as a past Certified Driver Rehabilitation Specialist and for therapeutic use of Interactive Metronome to treat processing disorders.

Ileana has served as an expert witness for cases involving infants and children. She is a published author in the areas of case management and life care planning, as well as energy conservation, motion economy, sleep issues for children with Autism and other Sensory Processing Disorders, and interventions related to clinical and school-based pediatric practice. She collaborated in a research study in 2009 with the graduate level O.T. students at Brenau University that was based on a therapy tool she published called, The Scale of Sensory Strategies (S.O.S.S.)®ToolKit. She has authored five other publications with the book prior to this one entitled, AUTISM SLEEPS: Sensory Strategies to Help Restless Minds Sleep.

Having presented inservices, seminars and workshops throughout her career, Ileana is an experienced speaker. She has covered subject matters from the Neonatal Intensive Care Unit to pediatric concerns in the home, school and community, especially with regards to sensory strategy implementation for a variety of behavioral concerns and disabled driver rehabilitation for adolescents and adults. Since 2010 she has been presenting a series of seminars across the country on how to develop an evidence-based sensory strategy plan to treat sensory-based problem behaviors.

Ileana was honored at the Medical College of Georgia where she was given the Barbara S. Grant Award from the Georgia O.T. Association in October 2005 for her dedication and lifetime of outstanding service to the field of occupational therapy. In 1977 she received the Maddak Award in the area of Physical Disability for the design of the *S.K.A.T.E.* (Skateboard for Kinesthetic Arm Therapeutic Exercises).

Among her most meaningful accomplishments, she is credited with implementing the first Neonatal ICU Occupational Therapy program in Georgia at DeKalb Medical Center in 1979. She was also the first Occupational Therapist to develop and implement services at Scottish Rite Children's hospital in 1981, and established the first private practice Disabled Driver Rehabilitation program in Georgia in 1982.

Ileana retired from the Gwinnett County Public Schools after twenty years of service in 2015. She continued her work in school systems with Barrow County public schools, serving elementary, middle and high schools in the Special Education Department for the next school year. She provided Related Services for direct and consultative support to teachers and special needs students to help meet their Individualized Education Plan objectives. Since 2016 she has worked in two private pediatric clinics and in cyber school based services, providing home and community-based treatments as needed. As a wellness consultant and holistic therapist, she also incorporates alternative treatments as appropriate.

With a son who is a graduate of the University of Georgia, and a daughter with special needs who is an honors graduate of Kennesaw State University, Ileana is most proud of her children. She was born in Havana, Cuba, and immigrated into the United States in 1957. She is bilingual and fluent in English as well as Spanish, her native language.

Made in the USA
Columbia, SC
30 June 2017